Surviving
on the Foods and Water from Alaska's Southern Shores

THIRD EDITION

Dolly Garza

Published by Alaska Sea Grant

MAB-38   Price $7.50

Elmer E. Rasmuson Library Cataloging-in-Publication Data

Garza, Dolly A.

Surviving on the foods and water from Alaska's southern shores (MAB-38)

    1. Survival skills—Alaska. 2. Wilderness survival—Alaska. I. Alaska Sea Grant College Program. II. Title. III. Series: Marine advisory bulletin ; no. 38.

GF86.G37

Third Edition 2013

ISBN 978-1-56612-174-3

Credits

Editing by Sue Keller, layout by Jen Gunderson, Alaska Sea Grant. Cover photo of young popweed by Dolly Garza; cover design by Brooks Pleninger. Illustrations on p. 7 and p. 20 are from Eric Hulten, Flora of Alaska and Neighboring Territories, © 1968 by the Board of Trustees of the Leland Stanford Jr. University. All rights reserved. Used with the permission of Stanford University Press, www.sup.org.

Published by the Alaska Sea Grant College Program, which is cooperatively supported by the U.S. Department of Commerce, NOAA Office of Sea Grant, grant no. NA06OAR4170013, project A/152-20 and A/161-01; and by the University of Alaska with state funds. The University of Alaska is an affirmative action/equal opportunity employer and educational institution.

Sea Grant is a unique partnership with public and private sectors combining research, education, and technology transfer for public service. This national network of universities meets changing environmental and economic needs of people in our coastal, ocean, and Great Lakes regions.

Alaska Sea Grant College Program
University of Alaska Fairbanks
Fairbanks, Alaska 99775-5040
Toll free (888) 789-0090
(907) 474-6707 • fax (907) 474-6285
alaskaseagrant.org

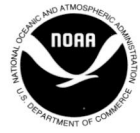
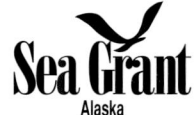

Table of Contents

ii	**The Author**
1	**Introduction**
2	**Human Body Requirements**
3	**Local Sources of Water and Edible Foods**
3	Water
6	Proteins
6	Carbohydrates
7	Fats
8	Vitamins and Minerals
9	**Preparation of Wild Foods**
10	Seasonal Foods
10	All-Season Foods
11	Edible Animals, Seaweeds, and Plants
18	Poisonous
19	**Non-Edible Animals and Plants**
19	Paralytic Shellfish Poisoning
20	Marine Animals
20	Plants
22	**Summary**
23	**References**
26	**Appendix: Nutritional Values of Wild Foods**
26	Nutritional value of edible sea animals
28	Nutritional value of edible wild land plants
30	Nutritional value of edible seaweeds

The author

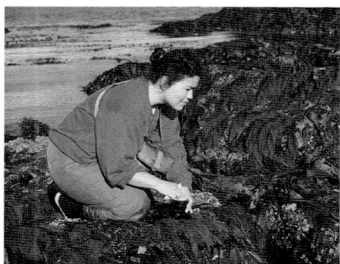

Author Dolly Garza on a seaweed-photographing expedition near Sitka, Alaska.

Dolly Garza has taught subsistence foods identification and use, as well as survival, in communities around Southeast Alaska since 1985. She grew up collecting and using subsistence foods with her family in Ketchikan and Craig. Garza is emeritus professor of fisheries at the University of Alaska Fairbanks. She earned her Ph.D. in marine policy from the University of Delaware.

Introduction

This booklet is useful to hikers, hunters, fishermen, recreational boaters, and other travelers who could get lost along the Gulf of Alaska coast. While it focuses on wild edible foods you can find along the eastern shores of the Gulf of Alaska, many of the beach foods are also found along the western shores of the gulf. The booklet provides basic information on edible coastal foods and obtaining safe drinking water. Whether you've gone high and dry with your skiff and are marooned overnight, or you've lost your way back to camp from an upper muskeg, the information on edible wild foods may sustain your body and mind overnight or for a few days.

In a survival situation wild edible foods may be the mainstay of your diet. While most people in need of rescue are found within 24 to 72 hours, rescue is not guaranteed and some people have spent days and weeks in a survival situation. Thus some knowledge of local wild foods is recommended.

It is also best if you (a) know the Seven Steps to Survival (Garza 1993; AMSEA, www.amsea.org), (b) have rudimentary survival knowledge, and (c) have a mental plan for spending the night with few or no provisions. Water and food are not the top priorities in a survival situation. It is more important to minimize heat loss to stave off hypothermia, and to set up passive and active signals so that rescuers can find you.

Most people who find themselves lost or marooned have few, if any, provisions. The stored gallon of water and coffee can of emergency rations will probably be on your boat or at your campsite, and not with you. What you are carrying with you at the time is probably all you will have to make do with. Once you have recognized you're in trouble (step 1), inventoried your supplies (step 2), minimized the heat loss from your body (step

7 Steps to SURVIVAL

1. Recognition
2. Inventory
3. Shelter
4. Signals
5. Water
6. Food
7. Play

3), and set up signals (step 4), you are ready to move on to meeting your body's needs. For optimum personal performance during the wait for rescue, the two most important essentials are (a) to consume adequate amounts of safe water and (b) to consume calories.

It is important to know safe sources of water and local wild foods. By harvesting, using, and preserving local foods for home use you are learning the what, where, when, and how of harvesting various wild foods.

Caution should be taken while learning to use local wild foods, as there are several poisonous and unpalatable plants and animals. Knowing and understanding the nutritional content of wild foods is not critical for short-term survival. But if you enjoy harvesting and consuming wild foods your knowledge could pay off should you find yourself in a survival situation.

Rescue often occurs in less than 48 hours, and you could likely survive without eating any foods at all during that time. However, food is a comfort to all of us and the act of harvesting, preparing, and eating wild foods may keep you occupied and in good spirits while you await rescue.

Human Body Requirements

In a survival (or any) situation, nutrients are essential for

- Energy for activity or heat
- Resistance to infection and disease
- Tissue repair
- Brain power and proper mental functioning
- Comfort and a feeling of well-being
- Body process regulation

Factors that affect a person's daily nutritional needs include stress, physical activity, exposure to the cold, and metabolism. The six groups of nutrients essential to proper body functioning are water, carbohydrates, fats, proteins, vitamins, and minerals.

Water is vital for almost all body functions including metabolism and digestion. Carbohydrates, fats, and proteins are sources of energy for the body, supplying necessary fuel for body heat and work. Vitamins and minerals are important in small quantities for various bodily functions.

Local Sources of Water and Edible Foods

Alaska Natives developed elaborate cultures based on regional fish, wildlife, and other natural resources. They learned safe sources of water and food, and learned to use local resources to create homes, tools, and clothes. During early times, experience served as the educator in learning the difference between safe and poisonous foods. Many of these foods are still collected and preserved using age-old methods. These cultures flourished over centuries, and today Alaska Natives still use many traditional foods and resources in cultural activities.

Alaska has a multitude of plants and animals. While it is possible to live off these resources, you must first acquire an appreciation for the edible and a respect for the non-edible or poisonous plants and animals. Familiarize yourself with the local resources by harvesting and eating them, to be better prepared to satisfy your food and caloric requirements in a survival situation.

WATER

Water is the most important nutrient, accounting for approximately two-thirds of the body's total weight. Water is involved in nearly every body process including digestion, absorption, circulation, and excretion. On the average, the adult body uses three quarts of water per day. A sedentary person may use only one quart per day, while an active person may consume several quarts per day. Water is lost through digestion, body waste removal, respiration, and perspiration.

If you continue to function without resupplying your body with water, you will

---

Survival Food and Water BASICS

1 In a survival situation, securing a safe source of drinking water is the most important nutritional requirement. Our bodies can go for weeks without food, but only days without water.

2 Know one or two safe plants or animals to eat during every season.

3 Finally, you should know which plants and animals are poisonous. As a rule: **If you don't know it, don't eat it!**

become dehydrated. Moderate dehydration can result in diminished functioning and mental dullness, while severe dehydration can result in death.

Symptoms of dehydration include

- Thirst (an initial sign)
- Headache (an initial sign)
- Dark urine
- Craving for cold wet foods
- Chapped lips and dry skin
- Nausea
- Dull mental function
- Leg cramps
- Depression (a killer in a survival situation)

If you did not bring any bottled or packaged water with you, you need to look for safe, clean water. In the wild, fresh water is available in lakes, streams, springs, bogs, ice, snow, and rain. However, groundwater (all of the preceding except falling snow and rain) can be contaminated and make you sick.

Giardia or "beaver fever" is a serious illness caused by consuming contaminated water. Symptoms include a vague feeling of physical discomfort, cramps, excessive gas, and abdominal bloating (Centers for Disease Control). The symptoms of this disease may not show up for several weeks, a period longer than the average survival situation. However, getting giardia can have long-term negative effects on your health if it is undetected and untreated.

You can also get diarrhea from drinking water contaminated with bacteria. The diarrhea and abdominal cramps can strike within hours after drinking contaminated water. Diarrhea can result in dehydration, which could be fatal in a survival situation.

Safe sources of water, anywhere outdoors, include rainwater collected in a clean container, groundwater that has been through a 1 micron pump-activated filter, and groundwater boiled for several minutes. All ground-collected water should be considered contaminated. It should be filtered, or boiled for at least two minutes to kill giardia parasites, and to kill diarrhea-causing bacteria. Store-bought chemicals such as household bleach, two percent iodine, and water treatment tablets

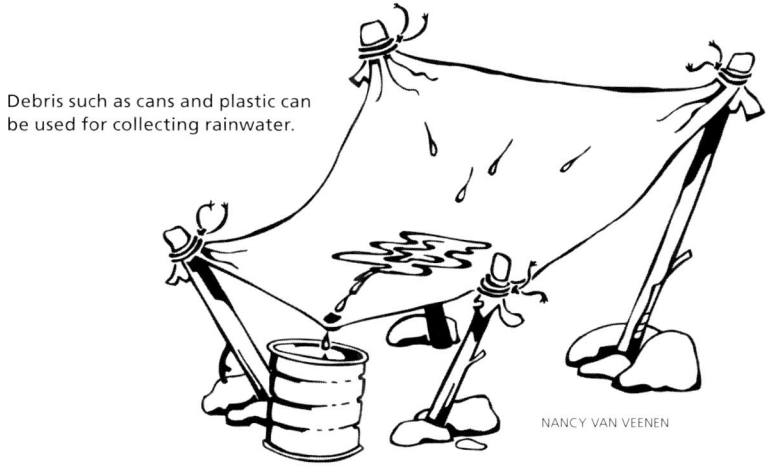

Debris such as cans and plastic can be used for collecting rainwater.

NANCY VAN VEENEN

may be used, but they are not 100 percent effective in killing harmful bacteria.

Finding clean containers to collect or boil water can be hard in a survival situation. Plastic, metal, peeled bark, large leaves such as skunk cabbage, and shells can be used for collecting water. However, boiling water may be difficult even if you are able to start a fire.

If you cannot boil water, and there is no rainwater, you should not consume potentially contaminated water. If you do not have a safe source of water, then limit your activities for the first 24 hours to minimize water loss while awaiting rescue. If you do not have a safe source of water and you spend more then 24 hours awaiting rescue, you need to be concerned about dehydration. Minimizing your activity and keeping warm will help reduce water loss from your body.

If you are able to secure safe drinking water, use your body as your water receptacle by drinking enough to quench your thirst. If safe drinking water is scarce, you need to limit what you eat because digestion uses water.

Do not drink salt water, which may make you sick and can further dehydration.

PROTEINS

Proteins are important for growth, development, and repair of body tissues and organs. The easiest proteins to obtain are shellfish and small fish. Avoid hunting animals, because you will probably waste a lot of time and energy stalking something you may not be successful in bagging.

Sea animals that you might find during low tide include limpets, small snails, chitons (gumboots), blennies (eel-like fish), small crabs, sea cucumbers, and sea urchins. Fish such as small flounder or rockfish can be caught near shore but may require experience as well as gear. Most intertidal invertebrates such as the limpets, small snails, and gumboots are slow movers and are easily harvested with a pocketknife or sharp-tipped shell or rock.

The protein content and species for some of the sea animals you may find are listed in Table 1 of the Appendix to this book. If you are stranded along the shore, proteins should be easy to secure and provide you with needed calories.

CARBOHYDRATES

Carbohydrates include sugar, starch, and fiber. Plants have carbohydrates in the berry, leaf, stalk, and root. Many of Alaska's plants are edible and nutritious. In non-survival situations some are harvested for fresh use, such as thimbleberries or fern fiddleheads, while others like beach asparagus or several of the berries are harvested and "put up" for winter consumption. There are several good references (Graham 1985, Schofield 1989, Turner 1995, Garibaldi 1999) that can help you get to know Alaska's edible plants.
Along the Gulf of Alaska, the more widely distributed species include licorice fern, wild celery, wild rose hips, salmonberries, cloudberries, currants, cranberries, blueberries, sourdock, fireweed, goose tongue, Labrador tea, and beach greens. Nutritional values and species of several plants are given in Table 2 of the Appendix.

Seaweeds also contain significant amounts of carbohydrates and proteins, although some of the carbohydrates are not digestible by humans. Seaweeds such as the bull kelp and several of the brown kelps can be found year-round. Other seaweeds including the black seaweed, sea lettuce, and dulse (ribbon seaweed) are seasonal and harvested during late spring or early summer (McConnaughy 1985,

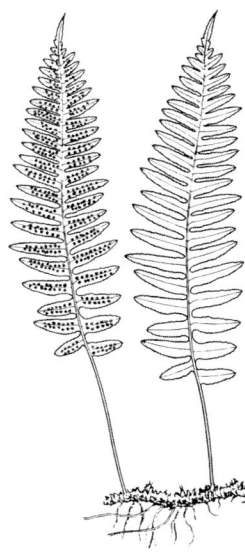

The rhizome (often referred to as a root) of the licorice fern has a high sugar content.

Druehl 2000, O'Clair and Lindstrom 2000, Garza 2005). Nutritional values of several seaweeds are listed in Table 3 of the Appendix.

Carbohydrates are more available from spring to fall and limited in the winter. Licorice fern and Labrador tea can both be found and used year-round. Licorice fern root has a high sugar content. The root can easily be pulled up from the moss and the outer bark peeled using your thumbnail. The root is a bitter sweet when eaten raw, and is often harvested and used as a medicinal tea.

FATS

Fats are the most concentrated source of energy in the diet, providing over twice as much energy as the same weight of carbohydrates and proteins. Wild sources of fat include sea urchin gonads, bird eggs, some fish eggs, and fatty fish including cod, herring, salmon, and meat. Sea urchins can be found year-round, at minus tides and in rocky areas with moderate to high wave action. Large animals and fish may be difficult to harvest in a survival situation, and few shellfish or intertidal life have significant levels of fat. Thus fat consumption may be limited in a survival diet. Proteins and carbohydrates should provide needed energy.

VITAMINS AND MINERALS

Vitamins and minerals are important in small quantities for metabolism, to help maintain the integrity of the skeletal system, and to serve as catalysts in biochemical reactions in the body. By consuming a wide variety of foods you will insure intake of vitamins and minerals essential to various body processes. In a survival situation consuming safe water and calories will be the priority, over critiquing foods for their vitamin content.

Seaweeds are good sources of vitamin A, vitamin C, the vitamin B complex, niacin, and calcium (Table 3 of Appendix), as well as iodine. The large and flat brown, red, and green seaweeds are all safe and can be eaten raw, cooked, or dried. Local edible and nutritious seaweeds include black seaweed, ribbon seaweed, popweed, winged kelp, brown kelps, bull kelp, and sea lettuce (Garza 2005). The vitamin and mineral content of these seaweeds is generally higher in spring and summer.

Most berries and greens have a fair amount of vitamins C and A (see Table 2 in Appendix). Excellent sources for vitamin C include rose hips, fireweed, cloudberries, cranberries, sourdock, willow shoots and leaves, and some seaweeds. Local sources of vitamin A include beach asparagus, fern fiddleheads, and sourdock. Good sources for the vitamin B complex, important for dealing with stress, are herring eggs, sea cucumbers, gumboots, crab, trout, black seaweed, bull kelp, winged kelp, fireweed, fern fiddleheads, and sourdock (see Tables 1-3 in Appendix). Iron can be found in good supply in seaweeds, gumboots, eulachon, and octopus.

Preparation of Wild Foods

There are several general rules for preparing foods in a survival situation. Seaweeds and almost all sea animals should be rinsed well in clean fresh water to minimize salt intake. However, if you do not have a safe source of water do not rinse foods. Because sea urchin gonads become mushy in fresh water, it is best not to rinse them at all. The gonads are eaten raw, or the entire animal can be laid on a bed of coals or a hot rock for a while to cook the gonads.

Edible leaves and berries can be eaten raw or cooked. Many roots are better boiled or roasted. Licorice fern root can be peeled and eaten fresh. Seaweeds can be eaten raw, roasted, boiled, or dried. Shellfish can be eaten raw, boiled, or placed on rocks near a fire to cook in their own shell. Fish should not be eaten raw, due to parasites, but can be boiled or roasted. To roast fish, wrap it in skunk cabbage leaves or large kelp fronds and place it on rocks near a fire.

ALL-SEASON Survival Chowder

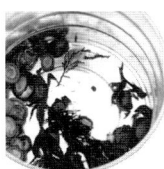

Survival chowder is an all-season nutritious and easy meal to fix using small intertidal animals, such as limpets or snails, and seaweeds. Use fresh water, not salt water. If you are using groundwater, boil the water for a minute. Toss in all foods, and boil for a few more minutes. The meat from the limpets and snails will separate from the shells. The water will be filled with vitamins and minerals from the seaweeds. Optional: add small fish or edible leaves or roots depending on availability.

Food Preparation

SEASONAL FOODS

Summer June–August

Chitons	boiled for a few minutes
Sea cucumbers	steamed or baked
Goose tongue and beach asparagus	steamed
Chickweed	raw as salad
Seaweeds: ribbon, brown, popweed, bull kelp	raw (rinse first)
Salmonberries, blueberries, and huckleberries	mix, for dessert

Fall September–November

Flatfish and blennies	boiled or steamed
Survival chowder; add Indian rice (bulbs of chocolate lily)	see previous page
Cranberries, currants, huckleberries	mix for dessert
Labrador tea leaves and rose hips	steep in hot water for tea

Winter December–February

Survival chowder; add Indian rice (bulbs of chocolate lily)	see previous page
Sea urchin gonads	raw or baked for 5 minutes
Wild potato (silverweed root, *Potentilla anserina*)	baked
Labrador tea leaves	steep in hot water for tea

Spring March–May

Small snails	steamed
Fern fiddleheads	steamed
Eulachon	boiled
Chickweed, willow, and fireweed greens	raw as salad
Herring eggs on kelp	raw or dipped in hot water
Seaweeds: ribbon, black, and sea lettuce	raw or boiled in survival chowder
Fireweed, young leaves	steep in hot water for tea

ALL-SEASON FOODS

Small snails
Limpets
Kelp (large flat brown seaweed)
Popweed
Licorice fern
Labrador tea leaves

Edible animals

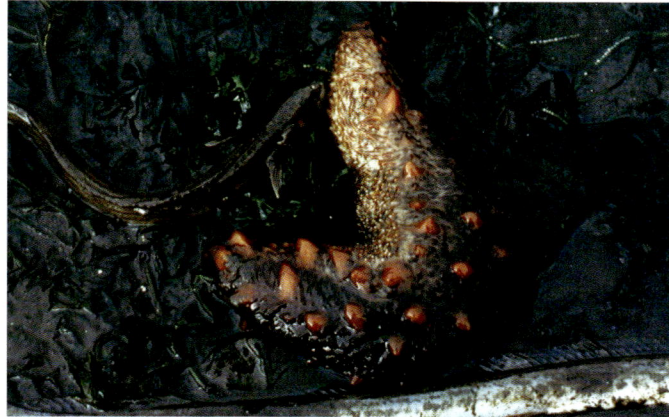

Blenny (left)
Sea cucumber (right)

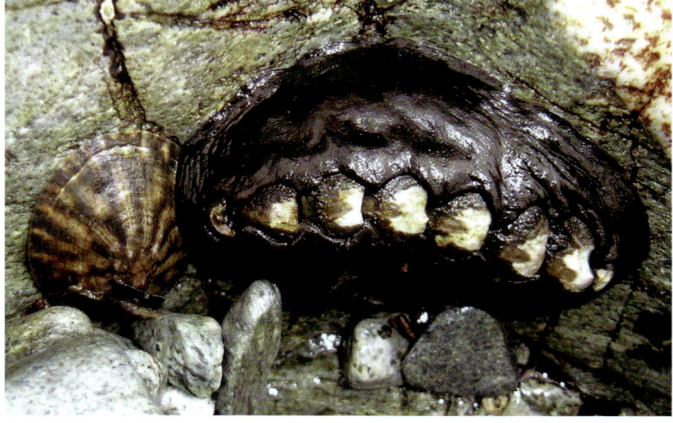

Limpet (left)
Chiton (right)

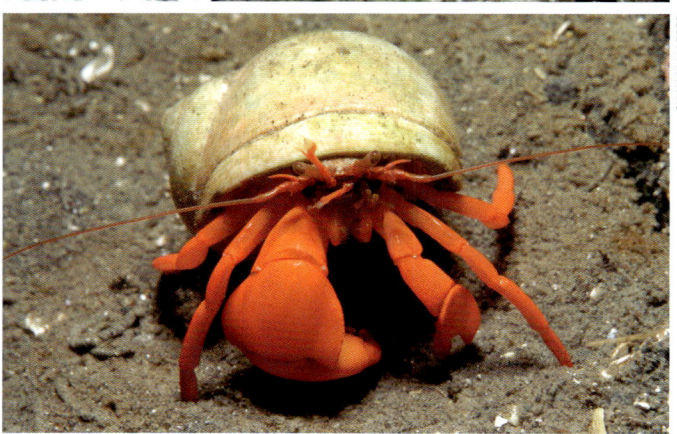

Hermit crab

Edible animals and seaweeds

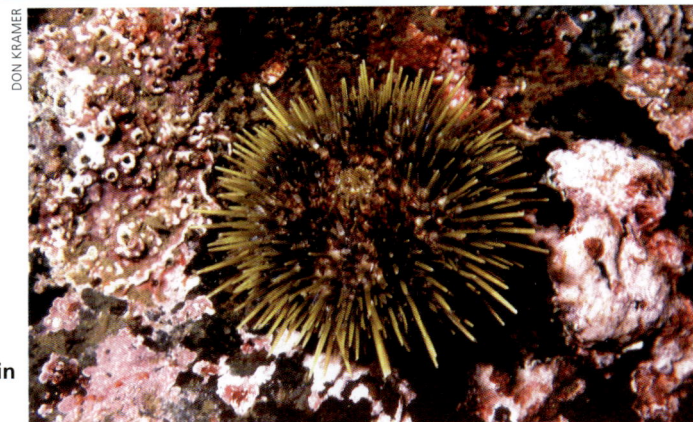

Sea Urchin

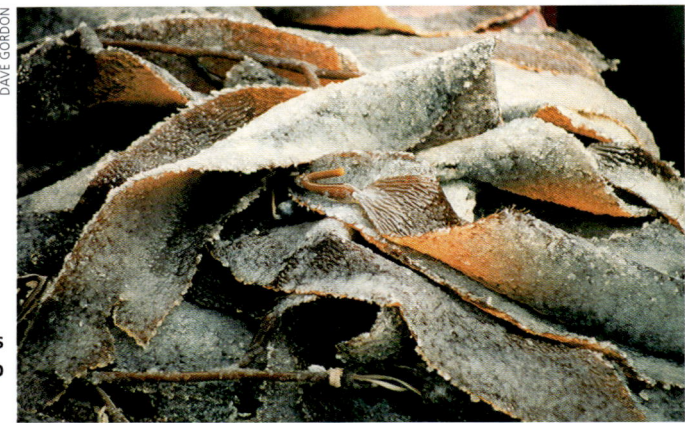

Herring eggs on kelp

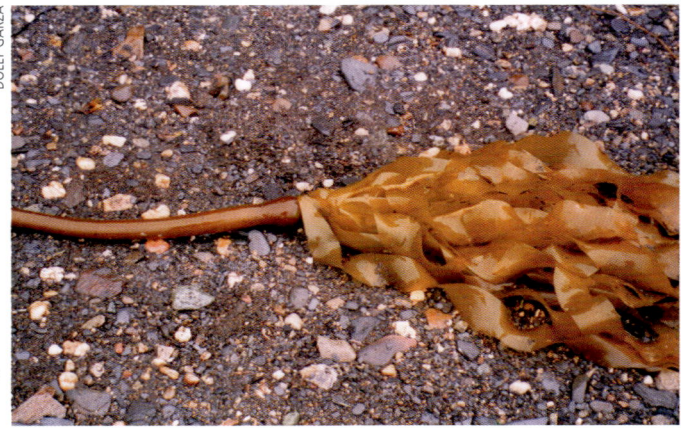

Bull kelp

Edible seaweeds

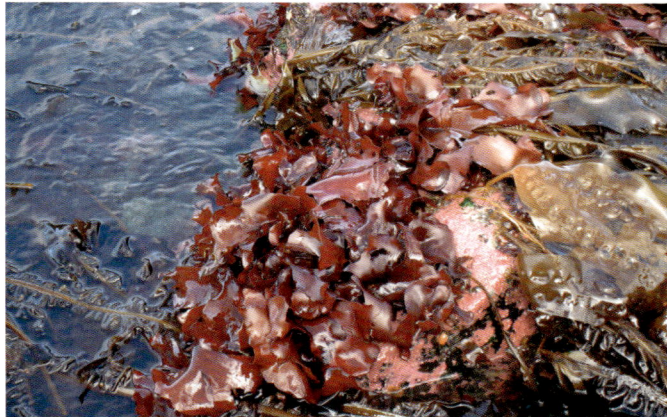

Ribbon seaweed

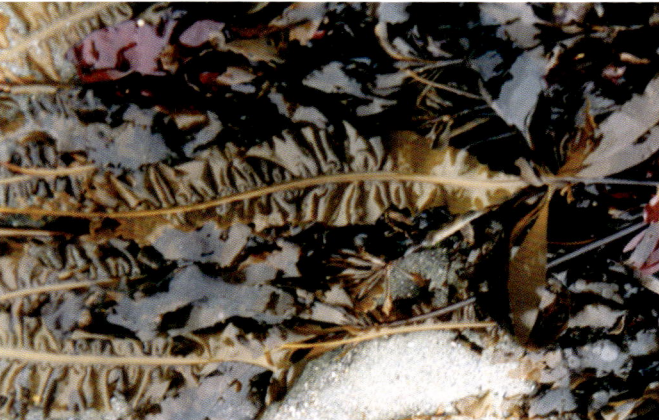

Winged kelp

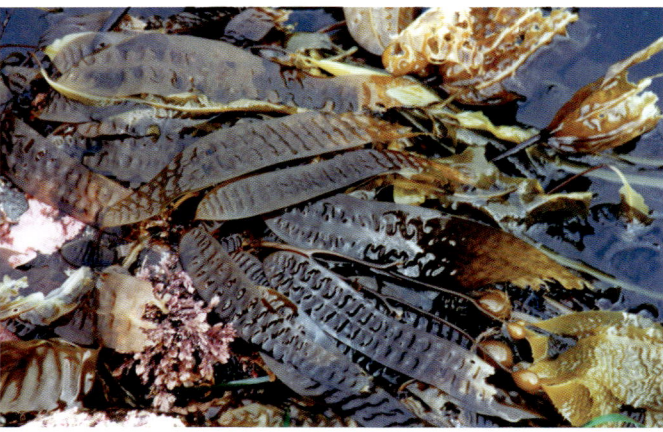

Kelp

Edible seaweeds and plants

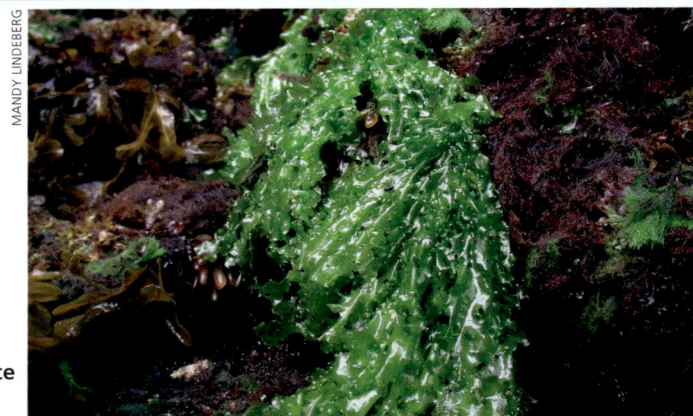

Sea lettuce

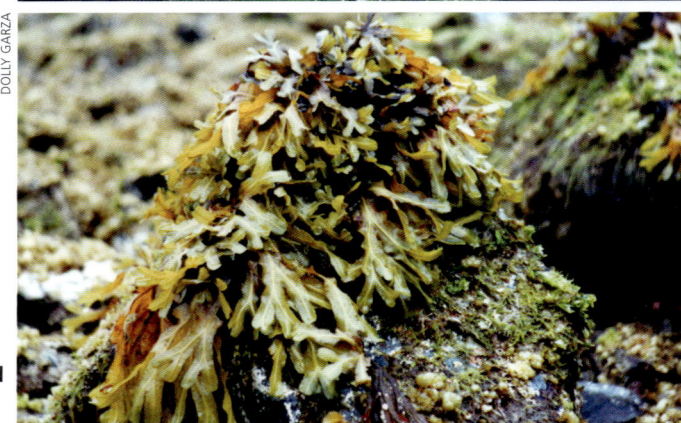

Popweed

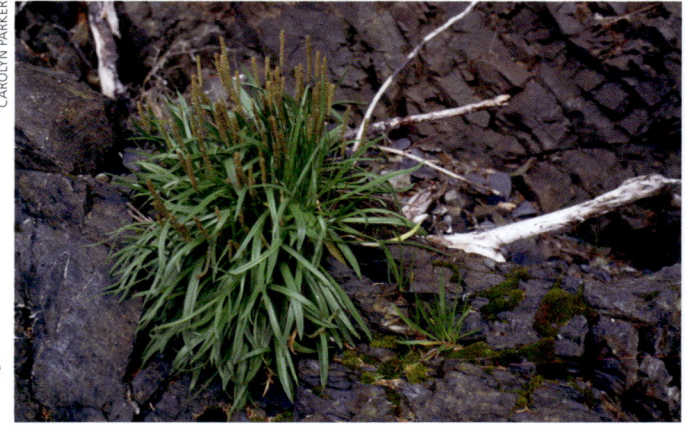

Goose tongue

Edible plants

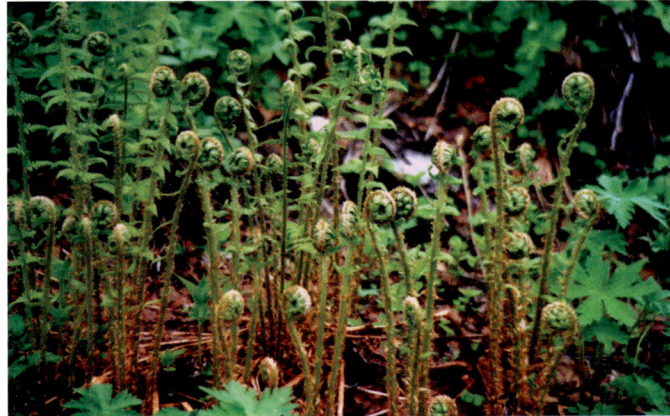

Fern fiddleheads

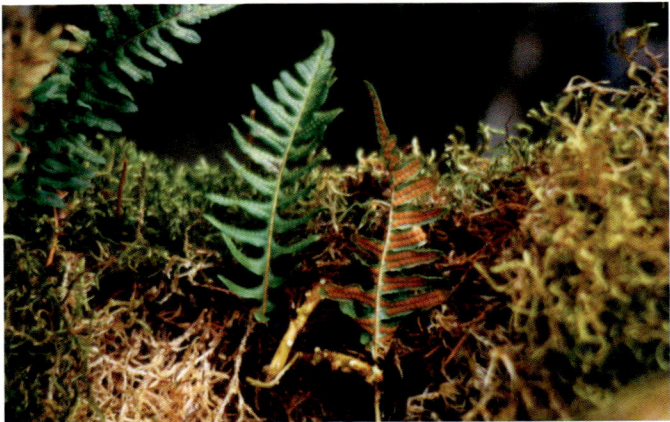

Licorice fern

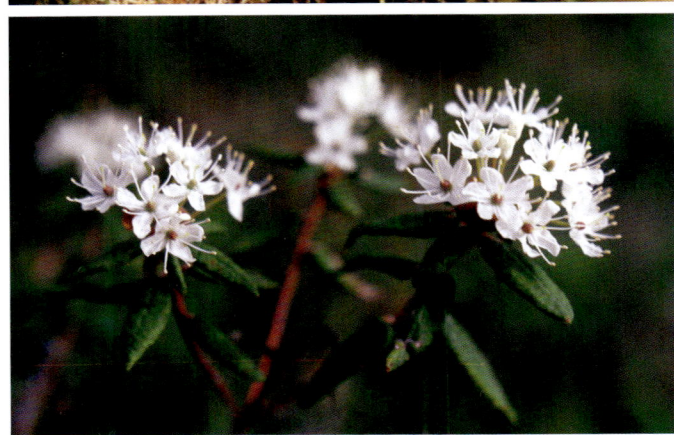

Labrador tea

Edible plants

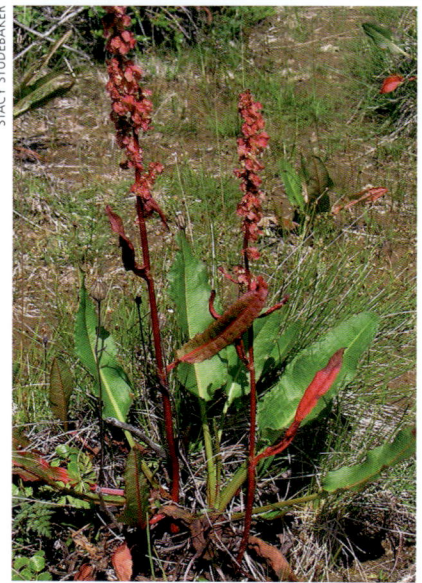

Sourdock

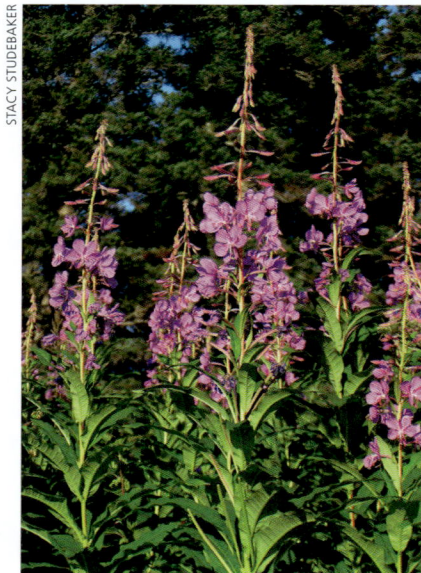

Fireweed

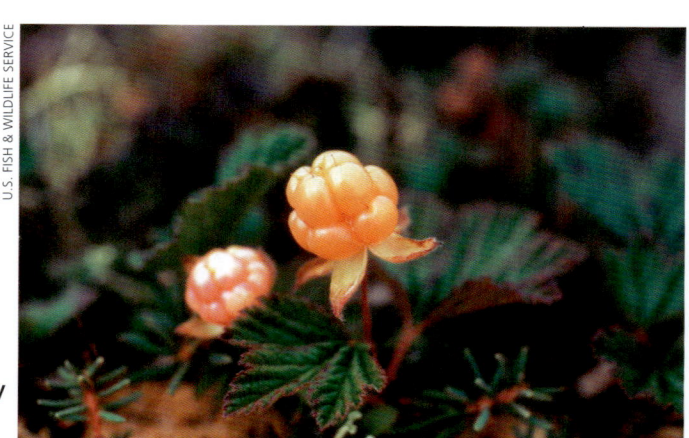

Cloudberry

Edible plants

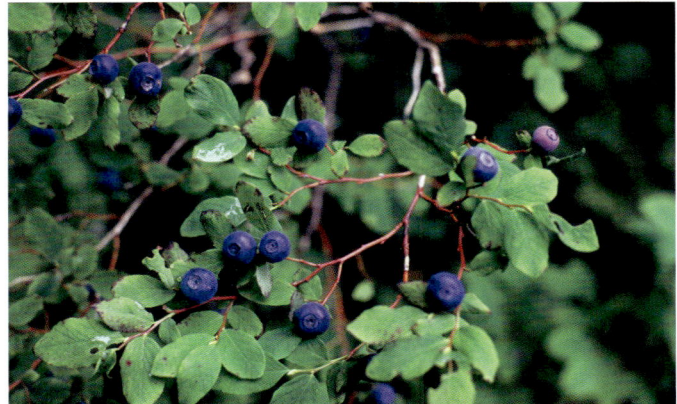

Blueberry

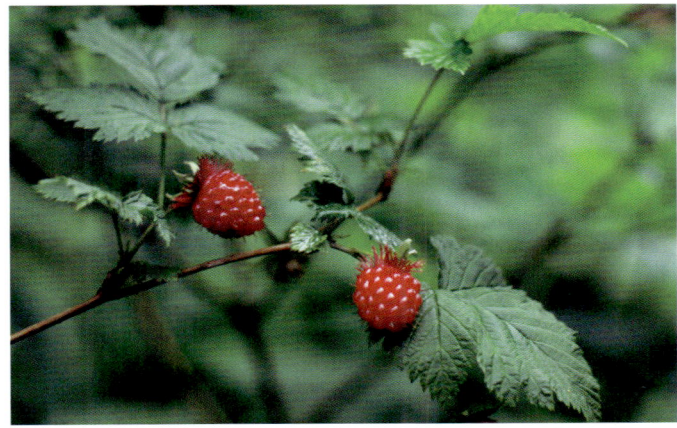

Salmonberry

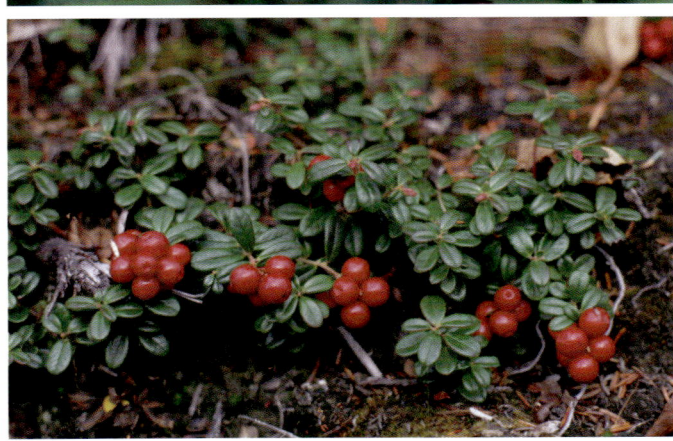

Lingonberry

POISONOUS

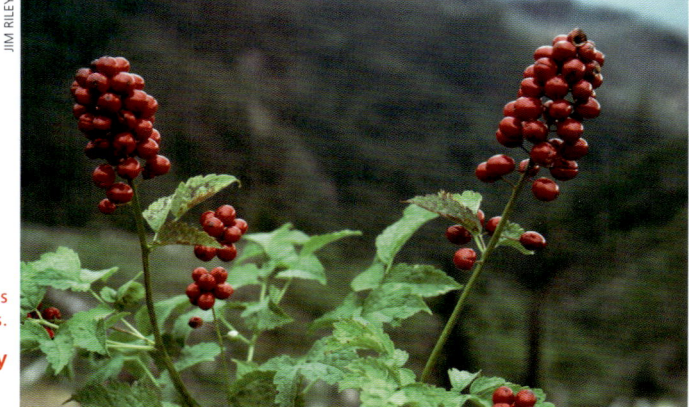

Roots and berries are poisonous.

Baneberry

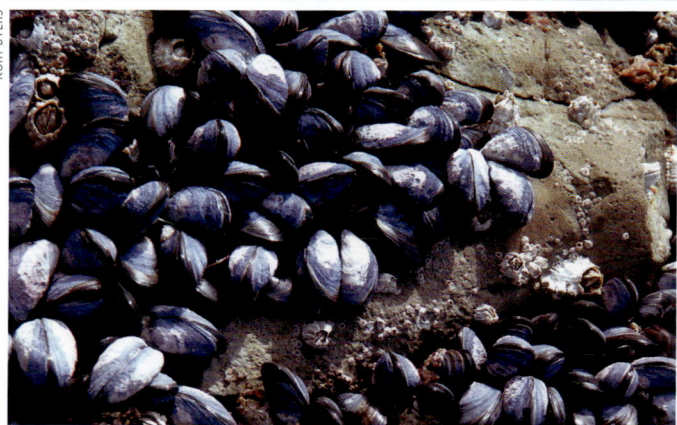

Mussels may contain PSP toxins.

Blue mussels

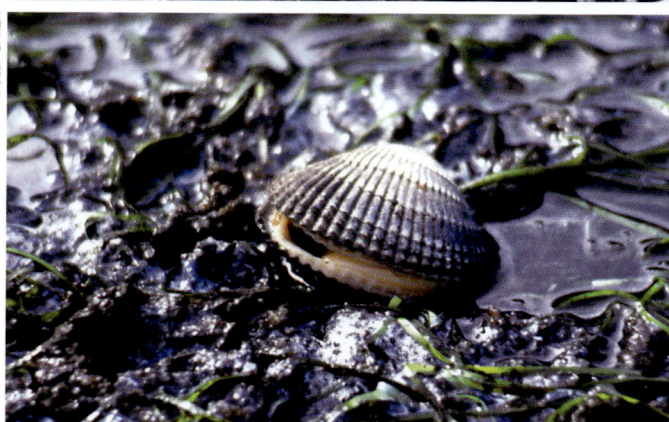

Cockle clams may contain PSP toxins.

Cockle clam

Non-Edible Animals and Plants
PARALYTIC SHELLFISH POISONING

All of the bivalve shellfish (shellfish with two shells) may contain saxitoxins that cause paralytic shellfish poisoning (PSP), hence are unsafe to eat in the wilderness (RaLonde 1996). PSP is caused by dinoflagellates with extremely potent neurotoxins that block nerve impulses. PSP can result in death due to respiratory failure. The toxic dinoflagellate blooms occur more commonly in late spring and summer, but they also occur during other times of the year. While toxic blooms can color the water red, often called a "red tide," shellfish can be very toxic in the complete absence of red colored water.

Avoid all bivalves including clams, cockles, mussels, scallops, oysters, and geoduck. Mussels can accumulate high levels of toxins and eating a handful of toxic mussels could lead to death.

In addition, filter-feeding barnacles and clam-eating moon snails have tested positive for these toxins. Bivalves accumulate different levels of PSP toxins, and the duration of the toxicity varies. The time it takes for shellfish to rid themselves of the toxins after a PSP "event" is unpredictable, and can last from weeks to years.

Even if you eat clams or other bivalves at home, do not eat them in a survival situation. If you get PSP from eating clams at home, you are probably able to get medical help. If you are out in the wilderness, medical help will not be available and you will likely die from respiratory failure several hours after eating toxic bivalves.

Symptoms of PSP will start between five and thirty minutes after eating poisoned bivalves, although it can be longer. A tingling or burning sensation around the lips, gums, and tongue is felt, followed by a prickly feeling or numbness in the fingers and toes. This sensation may spread within four to six hours through the arms, legs, and neck. Drowsiness, incoherence of speech, impaired vision, headache, staggering, and respiratory problems may follow. Without proper medical attention, death will occur from respiratory failure.

MARINE ANIMALS

The sea star, sea anemone, jellyfish, sponge, nudibranch, and sand dollar all may use light toxins to immobilize their prey. These animals have little or no nutritional value and should be avoided. While the California sea cucumber, *Parastichopus californicus*, is edible and palatable, the orange sea cucumber, *Cucumaria miniata*, has an unpalatable odor when raw or cooked. The hairy triton, a greenish deepwater snail with small brown fuzzy hairs, should be avoided. Since it is a deepwater species, you probably will not find it along the shore. The moon snail, as mentioned earlier, can contain paralytic shellfish poisoning. The moon snail drills holes in bivalves to suck the meat out of them, and can accumulate poisonous saxitoxins from shellfish. It is found at low tides along muddy beaches.

PLANTS

Several of Alaska's plants are poisonous or inedible, and it is therefore important to know the plants you are considering for food. If you are not sure what plant you have, do not eat it. There are several good Alaska plant books (Graham 1985, Viereck 1987, CES 1993, Turner 1995) that will help you identify poisonous plants. Some of Alaska's

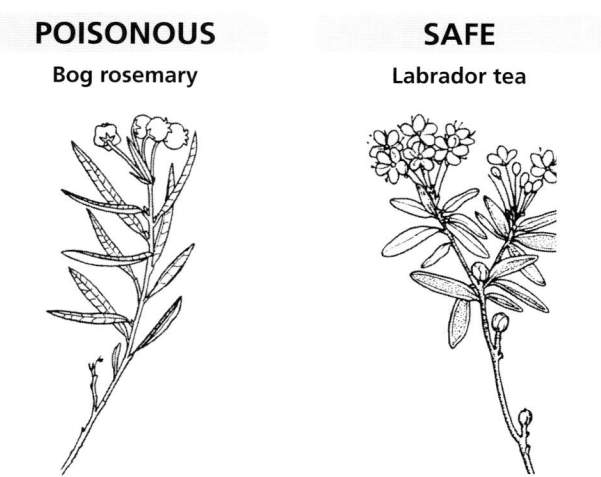

Bog rosemary and Labrador tea are poisonous/safe look-alikes.

toxic land plants are baneberry (it has red or white berries), wild sweet pea, water hemlock, narcissus-flowered anemone, nutka lupine, vetch, false hellebore, and death camas.

Several of the poisonous species of plants look similar to edible species. The poisonous water hemlock looks similar, and is related, to the edible and delicious wild celery, and can be confused with it (CES 1993). Wild celery is an important spring food to several Alaska Native tribes. Other look-alike poisonous/safe plants are baneberry/highbush cranberry, and bog rosemary/Labrador tea (Schofield 1989).

Labrador tea is a low bog bush that has leaves on it year-round. The leaves are oval shaped with a brownish fuzz on the underside. These leaves are packed with vitamin C and teas are made by Alaska Natives as a cold remedy. The flowers of this plant are white clusters.

Bog rosemary is similar in shape to Labrador tea, but has no fuzz on the underside of the leaf, and the flowers are small pink bells. These two plants grow in the same area and often side by side. Bog rosemary has a mild toxin that could make you sick.

Learn which plants are toxic before you began collecting plants as part of a family activity. Be sure you know the plant before eating it. Look for books and other materials that cover the edible plants in your area or take a class on local edible plants.

Two seaweeds to avoid include *Desmarestia ligulata* and *Corallina vancouveriensis*. The bright pink *Corallina* is a small, hard alga often found growing on rocks in exposed waters. Because these small algae look like coral and are found at a minus tide, it is unlikely that it would be used as a survival food.

Desmarestia ligulata is a large brown branch-like seaweed found in the lower part of the intertidal zone. When taken out of the water it often turns green, and when handled it will smell like rotten eggs. This seaweed contains sulfuric acid and is not edible.

While there are several edible delicious mushrooms found in Alaska there are also myriad mushrooms that should be avoided. Several species are known to be poisonous, and little is know about many other mushrooms.

Summary

Becoming familiar with the edible and non-edible land plants, seaweeds, and sea animals is a must for anyone who spends time in the out-of-doors and risks getting stranded in the wilderness without provisions.

This booklet gives basic information on nutritional needs of the human body and some wilderness sources to meet those needs. Water intake is most important to the body, and all surface water must be purified before drinking. It would be wise to carry packaged water with you. Sea animals from the intertidal zone are good sources of protein, and land plants are good sources of carbohydrates. Fats will likely be limited in a survival diet. Seaweeds and the berries and leaves of plants provide vitamins and minerals.

Some of the wild foods can be eaten raw and others can be prepared by boiling, steaming, or baking. In a survival situation, the season limits the foods and thus limits the recipes. Learn to identify and find one or two wild foods that you could eat in different environments and seasons.

Tables 1-3 of the Appendix list some plants and animals you can eat in the wilderness, and the reference section lists publications you can use to learn others. Find out about edibles by learning to identify them and harvesting them for home use. This knowledge can improve your chances of surviving a coastal emergency.

All bivalves should be avoided in the wilderness because of the possibility of paralytic shellfish poisoning, which can cause death. Several species of sea animals, seaweeds, and land plants should be learned and strictly avoided because they are poisonous. In a survival situation eat only what you know, and remember that rescue usually occurs in less then 48 hours.

References

Alaska Marine Safety Education Association (AMSEA). www.amsea.org.

Allen, M. et al. 2002. Surviving outdoor adventures, vol. 4: Small boat safety and survival. Grades 3-12. Alaska Sea Grant and Alaska Marine Safety Education Association. 262 pp. (Available at the National Sea Grant Library: nsgl.gso.uri.edu.)

Barr, L., and N. Barr. 1983. Under Alaskan seas. Alaska Northwest Publishing, Anchorage.

Byersdorfer, S.C., and L.J. Watson. 2010. Field guide to common marine fishes and invertebrates of Alaska. Alaska Sea Grant, University of Alaska Fairbanks. 360 pp.

Centers for Disease Control, Department of Health and Human Services. Giardia Infection, Fact Sheet. www.cdc.gov/ncidod/dpd/parasites/giardiasis/factsht_giardia.htm.

CES. 1980. Food energy and percentage of U.S. recommended daily allowance for eight nutrients provided by a specific amount of various foods. Cooperative Extension Service, University of Alaska Fairbanks.

CES. 1993. Wild edible and poisonous plants of Alaska. Cooperative Extension Service, University of Alaska Fairbanks.

DEC. Treating your water. Alaska Department of Environmental Conservation, Juneau. www.dec.state.ak.us/eh/dw/dwmain/Treat.htm.

Druehl, L. 2000. Pacific seaweeds: A guide to common seaweeds of the West Coast. Harbour Publishing, Madeira Park, British Columbia.

Garibaldi, A. 1999. Medicinal flora of the Alaska Natives. University of Alaska Anchorage, Alaska Natural Heritage Program.

Garza, D. 1993. Outdoor survival training for Alaska's youth: Instructor manual. Alaska Sea Grant, University of Alaska Fairbanks.

Garza, D. 2012. Common edible seaweeds in the Gulf of Alaska, 2nd edn. Alaska Sea Grant, University of Alaska Fairbanks.

Golodoff, S. 2003. Wildflowers of Unalaska Island. University of Alaska Press, Fairbanks.

Graham, F.K. 1985. Plant lore of an Alaskan island. Alaska Northwest Publishing, Anchorage.

Heller, C.A., and E.M. Scott. 1956-1961. The Alaska dietary survey. U.S. Department of Health, Education and Welfare, Arctic Health Research Center, Anchorage.

Hooper, H.M. 1982. Notes on nutrient analysis of several Southeast Alaska Native foods. Mt. Edgecumbe Hospital, Mt. Edgecumbe, Alaska.

Hooper, H.M. 1984. Nutrient analysis of twenty Southeast Alaska native foods. Alaska Native Magazine, Anchorage.

Hulten, E. 1968. Flora of Alaska and neighboring territories: A manual of the vascular plants. Stanford University Press.

Jones, A. 1983. Nauriat Niginaqtuat: Plants that we eat. Maniilaq Association, Kotzebue, Alaska.

Lindeberg, M.R., and S.C. Lindstrom. 2010. Field guide to seaweeds of Alaska. Alaska Sea Grant, University of Alaska Fairbanks. 192 pp.

McConnaughy, E. 1985. Sea vegetables. Naturegraph Publisher, Inc., Happy Camp, California.

Nettleton, J.A. 1985. Seafood nutrition. Osprey Books, Huntington, New York.

O'Clair, R., and S. Lindstrom. 2000. North Pacific seaweeds. Plant Press, Friday Harbor, Washington.

O'Clair, R., R.H. Armstrong, and R. Carstensen. 1997. The nature of Southeast Alaska: A guide to plants, animals, and habitats. 2nd edn. Alaska Northwest Books, Anchorage.

Pennington, H. 1986. Shore survival. Alaska Sea Grant Marine Advisory Program, University of Alaska Fairbanks.

Pill, V., and M. Furlong. 1985. Edible? Incredible! Landover Printing and Graphics, Seattle.

RaLonde, R. 1996. Paralytic shellfish poisoning. Alaska's Marine Resources 8(2):1-19. Alaska Sea Grant Marine Advisory Program, University of Alaska Fairbanks.

Schofield, J.J. 1989. Discovering wild plants: Alaska, western Canada, the Northwest. Alaska Northwest Books, Anchorage.

Schofield, J.J. 1993. Alaska's wild plants: A guide to Alaska's edible harvest. Alaska Northwest Books, Anchorage.

Turner. N.J. 1995. Food plants of Coastal First Peoples. UBC Press, Vancouver, British Columbia.

Viereck, E.G. 1987. Alaska's wilderness medicines: Healthful plants of the far north. Alaska Northwest Publishing, Anchorage.

Watt, B.K., and A.L. Merrill. 1975. Composition of foods. Agricultural Handbook No. 8, U.S.D.A. Consumer and Food Economics Institute, Agricultural Research Service, Washington, D.C.

World Health Organization. 1984. Aquatic (marine and freshwater) biotoxins. Environmental Health Criteria 37, Geneva, Switzerland.

Appendix
NUTRITIONAL VALUES OF WILD FOODS

Table 1. Nutritional value of edible sea animals, per 100 grams.

Name	Reference	Calories	Protein (g)	Fat (g)
Abalone (*Haliotis kamtschatkana*)	CES 1980	98	18.70	0.5
Chiton (gumboots) (*Katharina tunicata*)	Hooper 1984	83	17.10	1.6
Crab, Dungeness (*Cancer magister*)	Watt and Merrill 1975	93	17.30	1.9
Eulachon, raw (*Thaleichthys pacificus*)	Watt and Merrill 1975	118	14.60	6.2
Flounder, baked	Watt and Merrill 1975	202	30.00	8.2
Halibut, Pacific (*Hippoglossus stenolepis*)	Watt and Merrill 1975	171	25.20	7.0
Herring eggs on kelp (*Macrocystis integrifolia*)	Hooper 1984	59	11.30	0.8
Herring eggs, plain (*Clupia pallasii*)	Hooper 1984	56	9.6	1.0
Herring, Pacific (*Clupea pallasii*)	Watt and Merrill 1975	98	17.50	2.6
Needlefish (*Pungitius pungitius*)	Heller and Scott 1956-61		9.90	6.2
Octopus (*Octopus dofleini*)	Hooper 1984	57	11.90	0.6
Pink shrimp	Watt and Merrill 1975	91	18.10	0.8
Salmon, pink raw (*Oncorhynchus gorbuscha*)	Watt and Merrill 1975	119	20.00	3.7
Salmon, sockeye dried (*Oncorhynchus nerka*)	Hooper 1984	371	57.20	14.4
Sea cucumber (*Parastichopus californicus*)	Hooper 1984	68	13.00	0.4
Smelt (*Osmerus dentex*)	Heller and Scott 1956-61		16.50	5.1
Squid	Watt and Merrill 1975	84	16.40	0.90
Trout, rainbow (*Salmo gairdneri*)	Watt and Merrill 1975	195	21.50	11.4

Vitamin A (IU)	Vitamin C (mg)	Thiamine (mg)	Riboflavin (mg)	Niacin (mg)	Calcium (mg)	Iron (mg)
			0.18	0.14	37	2.40
1650		0.05	0.34	4.20	121	16.00
2170	2.00	0.16	0.08	2.80	43	0.80
			0.04	0.04		
	2.00	0.07	0.08	2.50	23	1.40
53	680.00	0.05	0.07	8.30	16	0.80
89		0.10	0.13	2.70	161	3.40
57	0.60	0.10	0.12	1.80	19	2.70
100	3.00	0.02	0.16	3.50		1.30
1230		0.05	1.38		93	5.00
		0.03	0.04	2.10	24	5.30
		0.02	0.03	3.20	63	1.60
		0.14	0.05			
355	0.02	0.14	0.60	20.20	136	1.90
310		0.05	0.94	3.20	30	0.60
460			0.13	1.50	74	0.60
		0.02	0.12		12	0.50
		0.08	0.20	8.40		

Table 2. Nutritional value of edible wild land plants, per 100 grams.

Name	Reference	Calories	Protein (g)	Fat (g)
Beach asparagus (*Salicornia pacifica*)	Hooper 1984	27	1.80	0.3
Blueberries (*Vaccinium* spp.)	Hooper 1984	44	0.70	
Buttercup leaves (*Ranunculus pallasi*)	Heller and Scott 1956-61		2.50	0.6
Cloudberry (*Rubus chamaemorus*)	Heller and Scott 1956-61		2.40	0.8
Cranberry	Heller and Scott 1956-61		0.40	0.5
Lady fern (*Athyrium filix-femina*)	Hooper 1984	34	3.20	0.2
Fireweed leaves (*Epilobium latifolium*)	Heller and Scott 1956-61		3.00	0.80
Goose tongue (*Plantago maritima*)	Hooper 1982			
Huckleberry (*Vaccinium parvifolium*)	Hooper 1984	37	0.40	0.1
Labrador tea (*Ledum palustre*)	Hooper 1982			
Lingonberry (*Vaccinium vitis-idaea*)			0.40	0.5
Salmonberry (*Rubus spectabilis*)	Hooper 1984	44	1.00	0.1
Sitka rose hips (*Rosa acicularis*)	Hooper 1982			
Sourdock (*Rumex arcticus*)	Heller and Scott 1956-61		2.30	0.7
Stonecrop (*Sedum roseum*)	Heller and Scott 1956-61		1.20	1.0
Willow (*Salix* spp.)	Heller and Scott 1956-61	33	6.10	

Vitamin A (IU)	Vitamin C (mg)	Thiamine (mg)	Riboflavin (mg)	Niacin (mg)	Calcium (mg)	Iron (mg)
1922	1.80	0.01	0.09	0.70	45	0.90
163	2.20	0.03	0.10	0.40	15	1.10
4840		0.04	0.69	1.20	11	2.90
210	158.00	0.05	0.07	0.90	18	0.70
90	21.00	0.02	0.08	0.40	26	0.40
1340	8.90	0.00	0.25	2.00	23	0.80
5720		0.04	0.86	1.40	13	2.10
	2.97			502.50	18	3.20
79	2.80	0.01	0.03	0.30	15	0.31
	0.30			131.80		
90		0.02	0.08	0.40	26	0.40
1550	2.40	0.04	0.07	0.10	14	0.64
	290.99			26.20		
11900	68.00	0.09	0.54	1.10	2	0.80
6250		0.03	0.34	0.80	1	0.60
18700	190.00			2.30	130	2.60

Table 3. Nutritional value of edible seaweeds, per 100 grams.

Name	Reference	Calories	Protein (g)	Fat (g)
Alaria (*Alaria*)	McConnaughy 1985		12.70	1.5
Black seaweed, dried (*Porphyra* sp.)	Hooper 1984	298	28.70	2.0
Bull kelp (*Nereocystis*)	McConnaughy 1985		7.30	1.1
Dulse, raw (*Dilsea edulis*)	McConnaughy 1985		25.30	3.2
Laminaria (*Laminaria*)	McConnaughy 1985		6.50	
Ribbon seaweed, dried (*Palmaria palmata*)	Hooper 1984	323	19.90	0.6
Sea lettuce (*Ulva*)	McConnaughy 1985		20.00	
Wakime (*Undaria*)	McConnaughy 1985		12.00	

Vitamin A (IU)	Vitamin C (mg)	Thiamine (mg)	Riboflavin (mg)	Niacin (mg)	Calcium (mg)	Iron (mg)
140	29.00	0.11	0.14	10.00	1300	13.00
4719	17.40	0.11	2.25	11.5	157	10.40
430	15.00	0.08	0.32	5.70	800	100.00
					567	
430	11.00	0.08	0.32	1.80	800	15.00
23	4.80	0.07	1.00	6.90	190	11.00
960	10.00	0.06	0.03	8.00	730	87.00
140	15.00	0.11	10.00	10.00	1300	13.00